Prasanna Venkatesan Eswaradass
Ramadoss Kalidoss

Evaluation of Central Neuropathy in Diabetes Mellitus

Prasanna Venkatesan Eswaradass
Ramadoss Kalidoss

Evaluation of Central Neuropathy in Diabetes Mellitus

Introduction,Objectives, Methodology, Review of literature, Results, Discussion and Conclusion

LAP LAMBERT Academic Publishing

Impressum / Imprint
Bibliografische Information der Deutschen Nationalbibliothek: Die Deutsche Nationalbibliothek verzeichnet diese Publikation in der Deutschen Nationalbibliografie; detaillierte bibliografische Daten sind im Internet über http://dnb.d-nb.de abrufbar.
Alle in diesem Buch genannten Marken und Produktnamen unterliegen warenzeichen-, marken- oder patentrechtlichem Schutz bzw. sind Warenzeichen oder eingetragene Warenzeichen der jeweiligen Inhaber. Die Wiedergabe von Marken, Produktnamen, Gebrauchsnamen, Handelsnamen, Warenbezeichnungen u.s.w. in diesem Werk berechtigt auch ohne besondere Kennzeichnung nicht zu der Annahme, dass solche Namen im Sinne der Warenzeichen- und Markenschutzgesetzgebung als frei zu betrachten wären und daher von jedermann benutzt werden dürften.

Bibliographic information published by the Deutsche Nationalbibliothek: The Deutsche Nationalbibliothek lists this publication in the Deutsche Nationalbibliografie; detailed bibliographic data are available in the Internet at http://dnb.d-nb.de.
Any brand names and product names mentioned in this book are subject to trademark, brand or patent protection and are trademarks or registered trademarks of their respective holders. The use of brand names, product names, common names, trade names, product descriptions etc. even without a particular marking in this work is in no way to be construed to mean that such names may be regarded as unrestricted in respect of trademark and brand protection legislation and could thus be used by anyone.

Coverbild / Cover image: www.ingimage.com

Verlag / Publisher:
LAP LAMBERT Academic Publishing
ist ein Imprint der / is a trademark of
OmniScriptum GmbH & Co. KG
Heinrich-Böcking-Str. 6-8, 66121 Saarbrücken, Deutschland / Germany
Email: info@lap-publishing.com

Herstellung: siehe letzte Seite /
Printed at: see last page
ISBN: 978-3-659-38546-9

Zugl. / Approved by: Coimbatore, Tamilnadu MGR Medical University, Dissertation., 2014

"EVALUATION OF CENTRAL NEUROPATHY IN DIABETES MELLITUS"

Dr. E. PRASANNA VENKATESAN MD DM

DR.K.RAMADOSS MD, DM

DEPARTMENT OF NEUROLOGY

PSG INSTITIUTE OF MEDICAL SCIENCES AND RESEASRCH

1

ACKNOWLEDGEMENT

With deep sense of gratitude, I sincerely express my thanks to **Dr. K. RAMADOSS,** Professor and Head, Department of Neurology, PSG Institute of Medical Sciences & Research, Coimbatore, for his valuable guidance and encouragement given at every stage of this project. I would also express my sincere thanks to **Dr.M.B.Pranesh, Dr.B.Prakash, Dr.G.Lakshminarayanan Dr.R.Balakrishnan and Dr.G.Gnana Shanmugham.**

I am very much obliged and grateful to **Dr. RAMALINGAM,** Principal, PSG Institute of Medical Sciences & Research, Coimbatore, for providing facilities in carrying out this project.

I am extremely thankful to all staff who have spent their time for collection of data and have also helped me in successful completion of this project. I thank **Mrs. SHERLY** and **Mr. SARAVANAN,** who helped me in recording the data.

I thanks my beloved parents for the confidence and encouragement given by them in doing this project.

CONTENTS

INTRODUCTION

Diabetes mellitus (DM) is a global pandemic affecting almost every organ in the body. It causes serious challenge to healthcare system. Nearly 150 million people throughout the world are affected and the incidence increases with time as sedentary lifestyle and obesity is on the rise. Major complications of DM are due to atherosclerosis and it can affect any organ in body especially eyes, peripheral nerves, kidney and heart. These are categorized into microvascular and macrovascular complications.

Diabetic peripheral neuropathy is a major public health burden. It is characterized by burning sensation of feet, distal weakness and absent deep tendon reflexes especially ankle jerk. Only 15% of DM have peripheral neuropathy clinically but upto 50% have peripheral neuropathy by nerve conduction studies. Similarly only 10% have peripheral neuropathy at time of diagnosis of DM but nearly 50% have neuropathy after 25 years duration. Duration of DM and glycemic control of DM are important factor for development of peripheral neuropathy.[1]

Various forms of peripheral neuropathy are known to occur in DM. The most common type is distal symmetric sensory polyneuropathy. Cranial neuropathies affecting oculomotor nerve, abducens nerve are also known to

4

occur. Rarely asymmetrical, painful proximal muscle weakness due to diabetic amyotrophy can occur. Only 0.6% of diabetic patients have optic nerve involvement resulting in optic atrophy.[2]

The peripheral nervous system involvement in DM has been studied extensively in various studies but central nervous system involvement in DM has not been studied in detail. The term "central neuropathy" has been unknown until recently. Only after few western studies described subclinical optic nerve involvement in DM by electrophysiological studies the term central neuropathy was recognized. Just like subclinical peripheral neuropathy, asymptomatic optic neuropathy or central neuropathy can occur and it is evaluated by visual evoked potentials. Although in diabetics the most common cause for blindness is diabetic retinopathy asymptomatic optic nerve dysfunction can occur as proved in various studies.

Visual evoked potential (VEP) is a non invasive, sensitive tool which measures the impulse conducted along the central nervous pathway. VEP measures the P100 latency which reflects the functional abnormalities of optic pathway even in early stages. We decided to evaluate the central neuropathy in DM patients and compare with controls. Although there were few similar studies in past most of them were in western literature and sample size were small. Hence we included larger sample size of 100 and we

5

also compared the latency prolongation with duration of DM, glycemic control and peripheral neuropathy.

AIMS AND OBJECTIVES

1. To compare the visual evoked potentials in type-2 Diabetes mellitus patients with that of healthy controls.

2. To find out if there is any correlation with duration of DM or glycemic control of Diabetes with P100 latency.

REVIEW OF LITERATURE

Diabetes mellitus (DM) is an metabolic disorder due to decreased insulin secretion or action or both resulting in hyperglycemia. It is one of the leading cause for blindness in world. It accounts for 30% of preventable blindness. The global prevalence of DM is 6.6% in 2010. As per international diabetes federation of 285 million diabetic subjects in world, 70 % live in low income countries like India. India is the diabetic capital of the world with 57 million people suffering as per 2010 data. If no drastic steps are taken to stop this epidemic it is expected to further increase in prevalence.

RISK FACTORS

1. Familial aggregation
2. Age
3. Adiposity
4. Body fat percentage
5. Insulin resistance
6. Life style changes due to urbanization
7. High prevalence of prediabetic condition

CHRONIC COMPLICATIONS OF DIABETES

Generally the injurious effects of DM are classified into microvascular and macrovascular complications.[3]

MICROVASCULAR COMPLICATIONS

1. Diabetic retinopathy

2. Diabetic nephropathy

3. Diabetic neuropathy

MACROVASCULAR COMPLICATIONS

1. Coronary artery disease

2. Cerebrovascular disease

3. Peripheral vascular disease

PATHOPHYSIOLOGY OF COMPLICATIONS

Although the precise mechanism for microvascular complications are not known it is generally believed that there are 3 pathways which are involved in development of these complications. It is related to both duration of DM and poor glycemic control of disease.

The central pathological mechanism in macrovascular disease is atherosclerosis. Atherosclerosis occurs in response to oxidization of LDL cholesterol resulting in endothelial injury and inflammation. Diabetes enhances the effect of other co-morbid conditions like hypertension, dyslipidemia, smoking and obesity. In addition there is also platelet adhesion, plasminogen activator inhibitor and increased free radical generation. All these factors collectively produce a state of hypercoagulability.

PATHWAYS INVOLVED:

1. Polyol pathway
2. AGE Pathway
3. Protein kinase C

POLYOL PATHWAY

In DM the excess glucose is shunted to aldose reductase pathway which results in sorbitol. Sorbitol is further metabolized to fructose. Neither sorbitol nor fructose can move out of the cell and it can result in cellular swelling. There is also depletion of myoinositol, loss of Na/K ATPase activity and NADPH co-factors. Hence the metabolically compromised axons are susceptible to injury and ischemia. The small thinly myelinated fibers are more affected than large fibers and hence sensory symptoms precedes development of motor neuropathy in DM.[3]

ADVANCED GLYCATION END PRODUCTS

Glycation of macromolecules in diabetes results in advance glycosylated end products. AGE are large aggregates and cannot be cleared by normal metabolism. They are susceptible to oxidation and resulting in oxidative damage. There is a very strong association between AGE and development of diabetic nephropathy. AGE is a complex series of poorly understood reactions in DM which results in endothelial dysfunction.[4]

PROTEIN KINASE C PATHWAY:

Chronic hyperglycemia in DM can stimulate protein kinase c pathway which mainly functions to alter vascular permeability, cellular proliferation and blood flow. Activation of this pathway leads to increase in VEGF and increased angiogenesis. This pathway has strong association with diabetic retinopathy.[5]

DIABETIC RETINOPATHY:

It is the most common microvascular complication of diabetes. It can even precede diagnosis of diabetes mellitus.[6]It is related to duration of diabetes and degree of hyperglycemia like most of the other microvascular complications. It is classified as proliferative and non proliferative diabetic retinopathy. The aldose reductase pathway and accumulation of AGE have been implicated in development of diabetic retinopathy.[7] In addition to blindness, diabetic retinopathy indicated end organ damage in a patient. Blindness in DM can be due to

1. Diabetic maculopathy due to ischemia or vitreo-macular traction

2. Proliferative diabetic retinopathy leading to vitreous hemorrhage or retinal detachment

3. Neovascular glaucoma

4. CRAO/CRVO (Central retinal artery/vein occlusion)

5. Ischaemic optic neuropathy

Strict diabetic control, regular ophthalmological evaluation and laser photocoagulation can prevent blindness due to diabetic retinopathy.

CLASSIFICATION OF DIABETIC RETINOPATHY:

1. Nonproliferative (background) retinopathy

    a. Simple background retinopathy

    b. Dot and blot hemorrhages

    c. Hard exudates

    d. Microaneurysms

    e. Macular edema

2. Prepoliferative retinopathy

    a. Soft exudates

    b. Intraretinal microvascular abnormalities (IRMA)

3. Proliferative retinopathy

    a. Neovascularization of the disc

    b. Neovascularization elsewhere in the retina

    c. Fibrovascular proliferation

    d. Vitreous hemorrhage

BACKGROUND VS PROLIFERATIVE RETINOPATHY

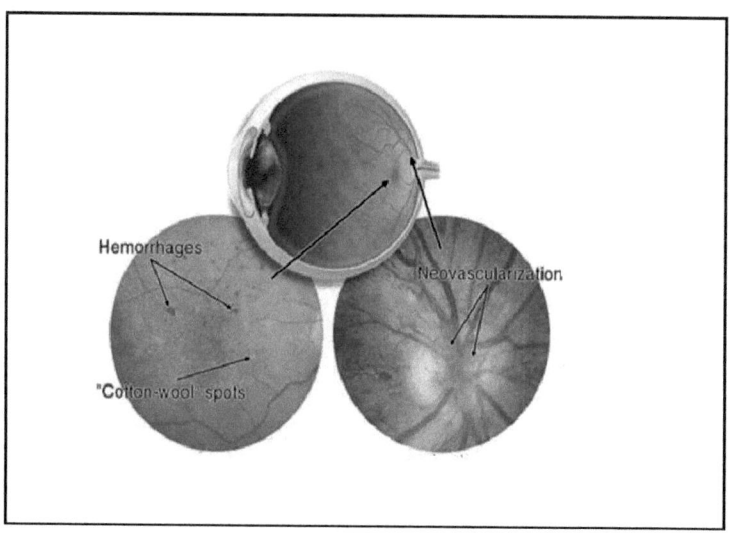

DIABETIC NEUROPATHY:

Diabetic neuropathy is a common microvascular complication occurring in genetically predisposed individuals in addition to longer duration of DM and poor glycemic control.[8] Recently there is association between sensory neuropathy and impaired fasting glucose without overt diabetes and persistent hyperglycemia with elevated HbA1c.

Both cranial and peripheral mono neuropathies which are of acute onset are mainly due to vasculopathy of ischemic origin. Pathologically there is ischemia of vasovasorum. The symmetrical distal polyneuropathy do not have evidence of vasculopathy. Hence alternative theory by Dyck proposed inflammation as possible cause. They found severe perivascular inflammation along nerve fascicles.[1]

CLASSIFICATION OF DIABETIC NEUROPATHY

1) **SYMMETRICAL**

   - Small fiber neuropathy

   - Large fiber neuropathy

   - Autonomic neuropathy

2) ASYMMETRICAL

   - Cranial mononeuropathies

   - Limb mononeuropathies

   - Lumbosacral plexopathies

   - Brachial plexopathies

3) PAINFUL NEUROPATHY

VISUAL EVOKED POTENTIAL (VEP):

VEPS are recorded from scalp as potential differences like EEG (electroencephalogram) in response to some visual stimuli. It checks the entire visual pathway and any lesion along the visual path can produce abnormal VEP. Its role in localization of lesion along visual pathway is only limited.[9] But it is very sensitive and reproducible test which can detect even subtle conduction defects in anterior visual pathway.

ANATOMICAL BASIS FOR VEP

The two optic nerves extends from retina to optic chiasm. Each optic nerve is about 5cm in length. At chiasm the temporal fibers remain uncrossed whereas the nasal fibers cross over and extend further as optic tract. They relay in lateral geniculate body of thalamus and from which arises optic radiation. The optic radiations terminates in striate occipital cortex (area 17).

Following activation of striate visual cortex, P100 waveform in VEP is generated. It primarily reflects the central field that is relayed to area 17. Peripheral retinal stimulation does not generate P100 waveform. The macular fibers which is responsible for central vision occupies large area in occipital cortex.

RECORDING VEPs:

Patient should be explained about the test and asked to sit comfortably in front of PC. Standard EEG electrodes are used for recording after degreasing the scalp. Electrodes Cz, Fz and Oz electrodes are placed as per 10-20 international system. Oz is active, Fz is reference and Cz is ground electrode.

1. Pattern shift VEP

2. LED goggles

In PSVEP black and white checks are displayed in PC and patient is instructed to look at center of checkerboard. Patient sits 100 cm from screen. Impedance is kept less than 5 kΩ. Average of about 100 epochs are taken so that VEP results can be reproduced.

VEP ABNORMALITIES

There are 3 types of abnormalities in VEP

1. Latency prolongation

2. Amplitude reduction

3. Both

RECORDING VEPs:

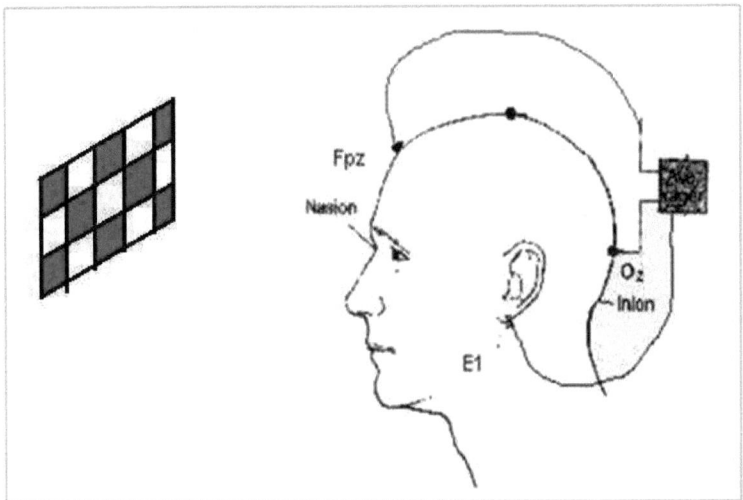

Fig 1: The patient is asked to fix his eye at the centre of the checkerboard which is flashed on front in a PC screen at a distance of 100 cms.

The commonest cause for P100 prolongation is demyelination of optic nerve. Unilateral P100 prolongation is likely prechiasmal lesion whereas bilateral P100 prolongation cannot be localized.

VARIABLES INFLUENCING VEP

1. **AGE:** As the age increases P100 latency prolongs due to age related changes. It was found that approximately 2.5ms prolongation occurs for every decade.

2. **GENDER:** Males have longer latency compared to females probably because of larger head and hormonal differences.

3. **EYE MOVEMENT:** Nystagmus, eye movements alter amplitude but not latency of P100.

4. **EYE DOMINANCE:** P100 latency is prolonged for non dominant eye compared to dominant eye.

5. **VISUAL ACUITY:** Only amplitude of P100 is affected with poor visual acuity and not latency.

6. **DRUGS:** When miotics are used for pupillary constriction they decrease the area of retinal stimulation and cause P100 latency prolongation. The opposite effect is seen with mydriatics.

7. **MENTAL ACTIVITY:** Arithmetic calculation can increase amplitude of P100 and decrease latency.[10]

CLINICAL APPLICATIONS OF VEP

1. DEMYELINATING DISEASES:

VEP is useful investigation in evaluation of multiple sclerosis. In patients with history of optic neuritis more than 90% have abnormal P100 latency prolongation. It is more sensitive than MRI in detecting abnormalities in optic pathway. Only 84% of symptomatic patients with MS show abnormalities in MRI. It can detect subclinical demyelinating plaque.[11]

2. OPTIC NEURITIS:

Typical optic neuritis is characterized by painful monocular vision loss usually occurring between 20 to 50 years of age. It is difficult to predict which of these patients with typical optic neuritis will develop MS later. Those with recurrent episodes and with typical MRI abnormalities have increased risk for developing MS.[12]

3. ISCHAEMIC OPTIC NEUROPATHY:

It is characterized by painless loss of vision usually occurring in elderly patients with vascular risk factors like DM and hypertension. It can also occur in vasculitis and giant cell arteritis. There may be altitudinal field defects. VEP study shows prolongation of P100 and decrease in amplitude.[13]

4. TOXIC OPTIC NEUROPATHY:

Some of toxins which can produce optic neuropathy and blindness are as follows

- Tobacco
- Alcohol
- Ethambutol
- Vigabatrin
- Amiodarone

can cause prolongation of P100 and decrease in amplitude in both eyes.[14,15]

5. NUTRITIONAL OPTIC NEUROPATHY:

Vitamin B12, vitamin E and thiamine deficiency can cause bilateral prolonged P100 latency.[16]

6. HEREDITARY AND DEGENERATIVE DISEASES:

Following neurodegenerative conditions can produce VEP abnormalities

- Friedrich ataxia

- Charcot Marie-Tooth disease

- Lebers hereditary optic atrophy

- Mitochondrial disease

Bilateral P100 prolongation is seen with normal amplitude. P100 prolongation usually correlates well with temporal pallor of disc.[17]

7. COMPRESSIVE LESIONS IN VISUAL PATHWAY:

Following lesions can compress the optic pathway

- Meningioma

- Tuberculoma

- Glioma

- Pituitary macroadenoma

- Craniopharyngioma

The extrinsic compression of optic pathway leads to P100 prolongation with drop in amplitude and distortion of wave.

8. CORTICAL BLINDNESS:

Cortical blindness due to bilateral lesion in primary visual cortex can produce P100 prolongation whereas bilateral lesion in visual association area with preserved primary visual cortex does not produce abnormality in VEP.[18]

9. MALINGERING:

VEP is very helpful in detecting hysterical blindness. A normal VEP in a patient complaining of blindness gives clue to diagnosis of malingering. But some patients can suppress VEP and cause P100 prolongation voluntarily.

10. INTRAOPERATIVE MONITORING:

VEP can be used intraoperatively while resecting tumors of optic pathway but has only limited role because of technical difficulties to provide proper illumination.

VEP RESULTS SHOWING P100:

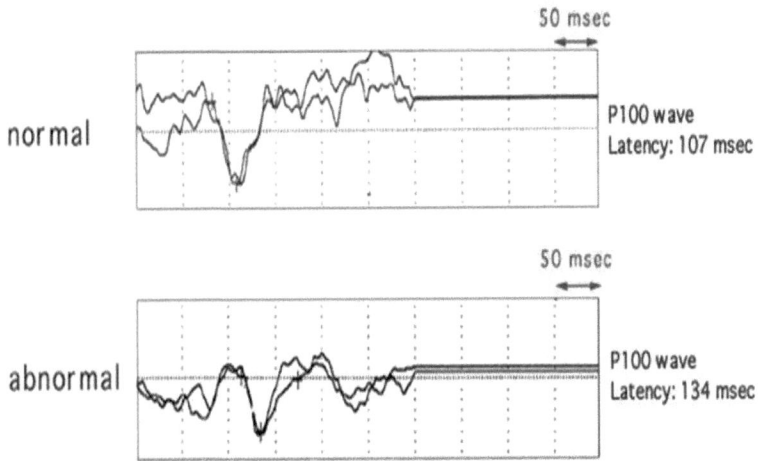

Ziegler et al in their study included 12 diabetic patients both type 1 and type 2. They subjected all patients to VEP and found that diabetic patients had P100 prolongation more than that of controls. The mean increase in P100 latency was 116.8+/- 4.5 with a p value <0.01. They treated the patients with continuous insulin infusion for a short period of 3 days. After 3 days of intensive blood sugar control VEP was repeated and they found that although P100 latency was slightly prolonged compared to controls there was significant reduction in latency compared to previous value. They concluded that P100 prolongation in diabetic patients were probably due to impaired glucose metabolism and is reversible with intensive glucose control for a short period.[19]

Dolu H et al studied electrophysiological characteristics of 51 patients with type 2 DM and compared with 30 age and sex matched controls. They did VEP, BAEP (brainstem auditory evoked potentials) and SEP (somatosensory evoked potentials) for all patients. The multimodal evoked potential which included VEP, BAEP and SEP were useful in evaluating central neuropathy. They concluded that there was significant latency prolongation suggestive of central neuropathy in diabetic patients compared to controls. They did subgroup analysis and found that latency prolongation in SEP, VEP, BAEP correlated well with duration of diabetes and not with glycemic control of disease.[20]

Comi G et al also studied multimodal evoked potentials in type 2 diabetes patients using VEP, BAEP and SEP. They found that central neuropathy due to cortical latency prolongation was more common in diabetic patients with peripheral neuropathy. Isolated abnormalities in VEP or BAEP or SEP was more common than all three getting affected together. They concluded that central neuropathy may occur due to hyperglycemia or hypoglycemia but exact cause is not known.[21]

Algan et al studied VEP in 50 type 1 diabetes and 19 type 2 diabetes. They found significant prolongation of P100 in diabetic patients with p value less than 0.001. But on further analysis they concluded that P100 prolongation did not correlate with duration of DM or glycemic control of disease. Their findings were contradictory to previous studies.[22]

Szabela DA et al studied 41 patients with type 2 diabetes. They recorded VEP in all patients and found 22% had abnormal P100 prolongation. They further analysed age, duration of DM and metabolic control of DM with P100 latency prolongation and concluded that there was no correlation with either of them.[23]

Again Szabela DA et al studied 50 patients with type 1 diabetes. They recorded VEP in all patients and found 26% had abnormal P100 prolongation. They further analysed age, duration of DM and metabolic control of DM with P100 latency prolongation and concluded that there was no correlation with either of them.[24]

Azal O et al studied 20 diabetic patients of which 6 were type 1 and remaining 14 were type 2. They recorded VEP in all cases and found significant increase in P100 latency in diabetic patients with p value <0.001. 45% of cases had P100 prolongation. They did not find any correlation with

27

metabolic control of DM or peripheral neuropathy. They concluded that P100 prolongation correlated well with duration of DM.[25]

Mariani E et al conducted a case control study which included 35 diabetic patients both type 1 and type2. They recorded VEP for all cases and controls. They found significant prolongation of P100 latency in cases compared to controls. They also concluded that P100 latency prolongation correlated well with duration of DM, HbA1c and presence of peripheral neuropathy.[26]

K Puvanendran et al studied 16 diabetic patients with VEP. They found 81% of cases had prolonged P100 latency compared to controls. They further analysed P100 latency with duration of DM and glycemic control of DM and found no significant correlation existed between them. They concluded that P100 latency prolongation correlated well with presence of diabetic sensory neuropathy.[27]

Yaltkaya K et al studied 25 cases of DM and controls. VEP was done to measure P100, N90 and N140. Sural nerve conduction studies were done to detect peripheral neuropathy. They found significant P100 and N90-140 interpeak latency prolongation. The latency prolongation correlated well with duration of DM but not with sural nerve conduction studies.[28]

MATERIALS AND METHODS

We conducted a prospective case control study in department of
neurology PSG institute of medical science and research from October 2011
to October 2013. Patients were chosen from neurology OPD.

INCLUSION CRITERIA

Newly diagnosed type 2 Diabetes mellitus and known case of DM were
included

WHO criteria was used for diagnosing DM;

1. Random plasma glucose of $\geq$ 11.1 mmol/l

   or

2. Fasting plasma glucose $\geq$ 7.0 mmol/l

   or

3. Two hour plasma glucose concentration $\geq$ 11.1 mmol/l two hours after
   75g anhydrous glucose in an oral glucose tolerance test (OGTT).[29]

EXCLUSION CRITERIA

1. Patients with long standing history of hypertension and with the past history of cerebrovascular accident.

2. Evidence of optic atrophy

3. Past history of optic neuritis

4. Visual acuity less than 6/18

5. Patients consuming > 100 ml of alcohol daily.

6. Patients with peripheral nervous system disease unrelated to diabetes mellitus.

7. Patients with diabetic retinopathy, cataract, glaucoma and vitreous hemorrhage.

8. Patients with type 1 diabetes mellitus.

CONSENT: Informed consent was obtained from patients who were willing to take part in the study. Ethical committee clearance was obtained.

METHODOLOGY:

50 diabetic patients who fulfilled the inclusion criteria were chosen and 50 age and sex matched controls were also included. They were subjected to detailed history to rule out stroke, past history of optic neuritis and other ophthalmological conditions. Detailed clinical examination, peripheral nervous system examination and ophthalmological evaluation including visual acuity, fundus examination was performed in all subjects. Later all patients were subjected to visual evoked potential test.

RECORDING TECHNIQUE:

VEPS were recorded using RMS EMG EP mark 2 machine with 2 channel and routine silver chloride disc electrodes. The PC based RMS machine was used and pattern reversal method was followed to record P100 latency. Before undergoing VEP, patient were instructed not to apply oil to head and take a shampoo bath. This is to decrease the impedance to less than 5Ω. They were advised not to use any mydriatics or meiotic 12 hours prior to VEP. If they use spectacles for refractory error they must continue to wear it during test. VEP is recorded in dark and quiet room. Patient sits comfortably in front of PC screen. Gentle cleaning of scalp is done before applying electrodes using spirit. Cz, Fz and Oz electrodes were used. Oz was active, Fz as reference and Cz was ground electrode. Fz is 12 cm above inion in frontal region, Cz in cetral area and Oz in posterior head region as per international 10-20 system.

The patient is asked to fix his eye at the centre of the checkerboard with checker of size 8*8cm which is flashed on front in a PC screen. The distance between the PC screen and the subject was kept at a constant distance of 100 cms. The aim was to achieve maximum stimulation of foveal and parafoveal fibers at 75% contrast and a reversal rate of 1.2 Hz. Uniocular stimulation was given separately for both eyes with white and black checks and the potential is recorded in wave form in a computer. VEP measurement normally produces a series of waveforms in PC which have negative and a positive component. The negative is N wave and positive is takes as P wave. The parameters usually recorded are P100, N70 and N155. Of these P100 is most important and it indicates latency of positive wave. They were measured in microvolts. Statistical analysis was done and p value was determined.

1. $p > 0.05$ (non significant)

2. $p < 0.05$ (significant)

3. $p < 0.001$ (highly significant)

WAVES IN VEP:

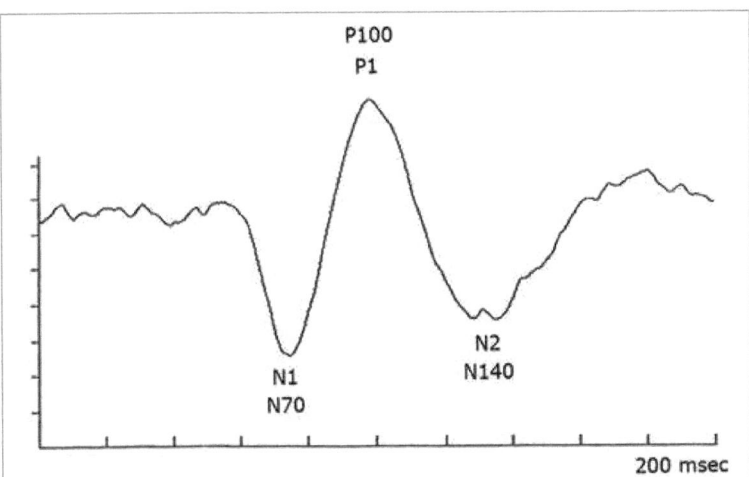

FIG 2: The time taken in milliseconds is marked in x-axis and the evoked potentials in microvolt are marked in y-axis. A graph is obtained with a positive peak PI00 and two negative peaks N70 and N155. The latency of P100 value is obtained and analyzed.

POSITIONING OF ELECTRODES

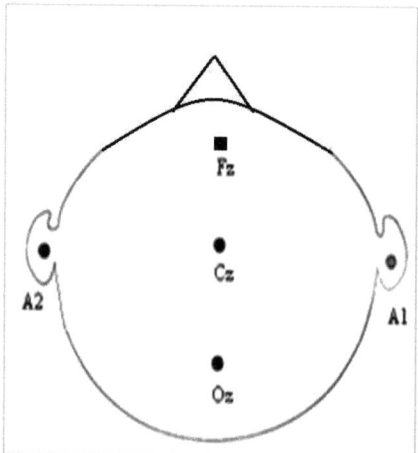

FIG 3: Oz -active, Fz -reference and Cz- ground electrode

OBSERVATION AND RESULTS

AGE DISTRIBUTION

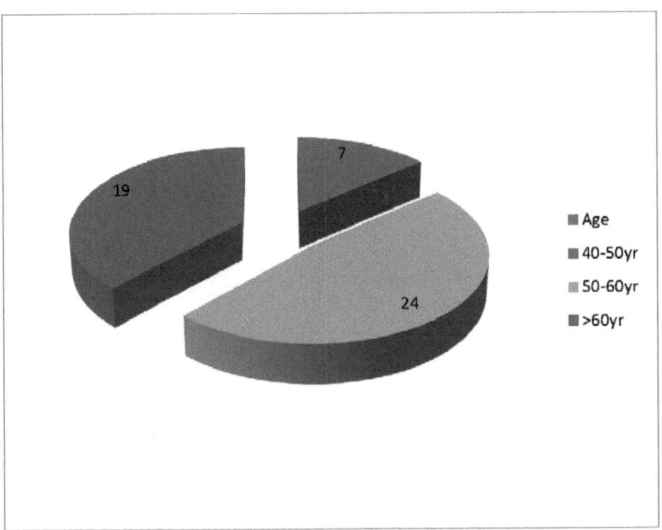

CHART-1: Shows 24 patients between 50 to 60 yrs, 7 patients between 40 to 50 years and 19 more than 60 yrs

SEX DISTRIBUTION

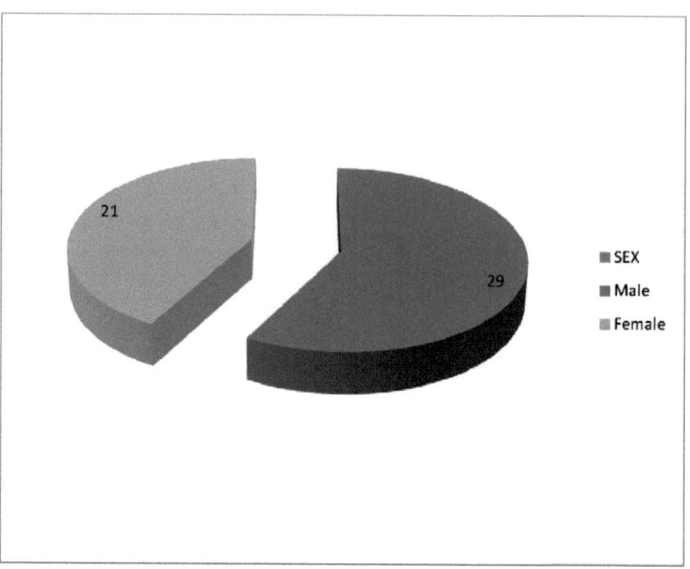

CHART-2: Shows 21 females and 29 males in study group

AGE VS P100

			Case P100		Total
			Normal	abnormal	
Age	Between 40 - 50 years	Count	2	5	7
(case)		% within Age (Case)	28.6%	71.4%	100.0%
		% within Case P100	22.2%	12.2%	14.0%
	Between 50 - 60 years	Count	6	18	24
		% within Age (Case)	25.0%	75.0%	100.0%
		% within Case P100	66.7%	43.9%	48.0%
	Above 60 years	Count	1	18	19
		% within Age (Case)	5.3%	94.7%	100.0%
		% within Case P100	11.1%	43.9%	38.0%
Total		Count	9	41	50
		% within Age (Case)	18.0%	82.0%	100.0%
		% within Case P100	100.0	100.0%	100.0%

AGE VS P100

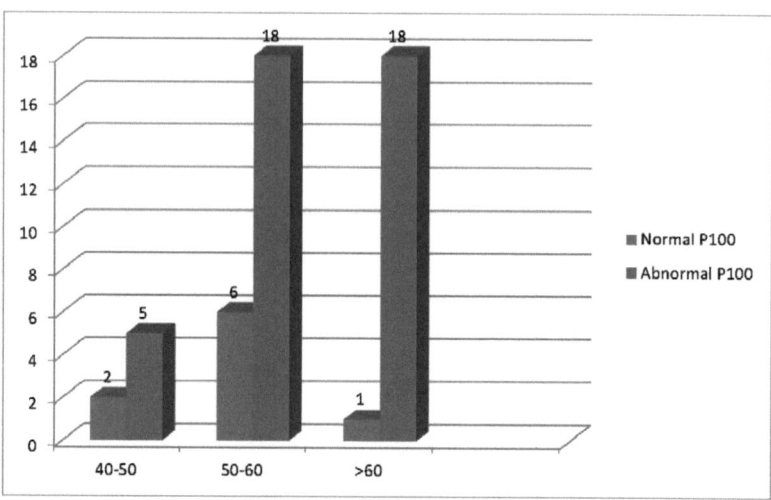

CHART-3: Among 7 cases in 40 -50 years group 5 had prolonged P100. In 50 -60 years group 18 had abnormal P100 and 6 had normal value. Above 60 years all except one had abnormal P100

SEX VS P100

			Case P100		Total
			Normal	Abnormal	
Sex (Case)	Male	Count	4	25	29
		% within Sex (Case)	13.8%	86.2%	100.0%
		% within Case P100	44.4%	61.0%	58.0%
	Female	Count	5	16	21
		% within Sex (Case)	23.8%	76.2%	100.0%
		% within Case P100	55.6%	39.0%	42.0%
Total		Count	9	41	50
		% within Sex (Case)	18.0%	82.0%	100.0%
		% within Case P100	100.0%	100.0%	100.0%

SEX VS P100

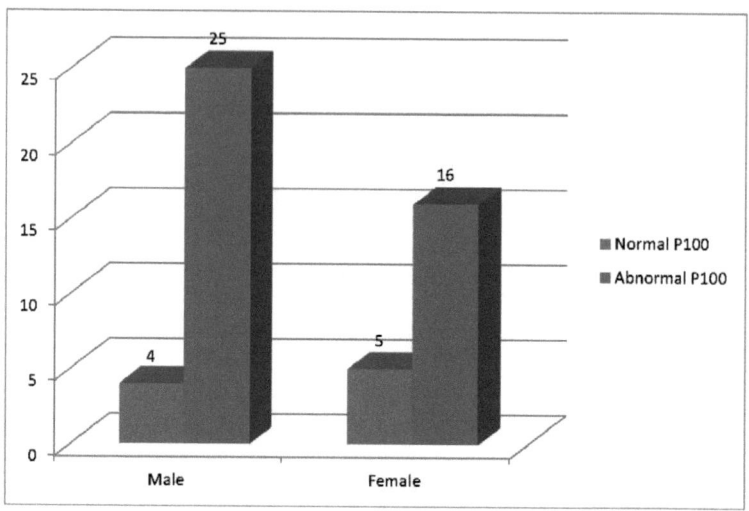

CHART-4: Among 29 males 25 had prolonged P100 and 4 had normal

value. In females 16 had P100 prolongation and 5 had normal P100.

CASE VS CONTROL

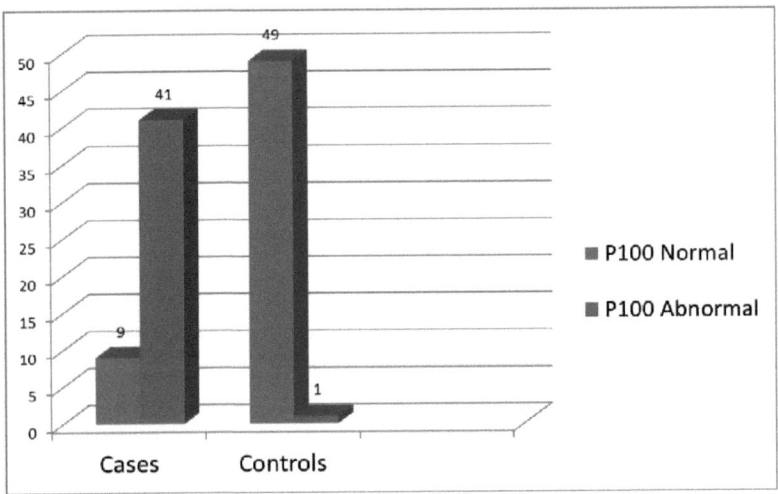

CHART-5: Among 50 cases 41 had prolonged P100 and 9 had normal P100 whereas in controls only one had prolonged P100 and rest 49 had normal P100

P100 VS HbA1c

Crosstab

			Case P100 Normal	Case P100 Abnormal	Total
HbA1c	Controlled	Count	5	15	20
		% within HbA1c	25.0%	75.0%	100.0%
		% within Case P100	55.6%	36.6%	40.0%
	Uncontrolled	Count	4	26	30
		% within HbA1c	13.3%	86.7%	100.0%
		% within Case P100	44.4%	63.4%	60.0%
Total		Count	9	41	50
		% within HbA1c	18.0%	82.0%	100.0%
		% within Case P100	100.0%	100.0%	100.0%

P100 VS HbA1c

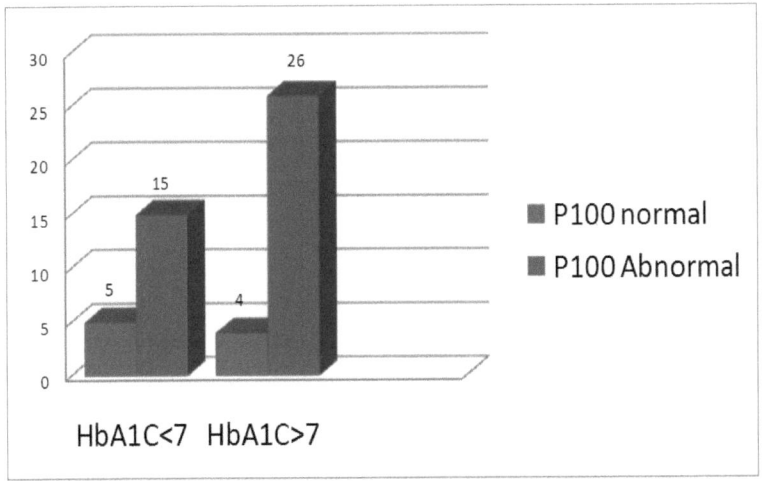

CHART-6: Among 20 cases with well controlled DM 15 had P100 prolongation and 5 had normal P100, whereas among those with uncontrolled DM 26 had prolonged P100

P100 VS DURATION

Crosstab

			Case P100 Normal	Case P100 Abnormal	Total
Duration	Less than 5	Count	8	12	20
		% within Duration	40.0%	60.0%	100.0%
		% within Case P100	88.9%	29.3%	40.0%
	5 - 10	Count	1	9	10
		% within Duration	10.0%	90.0%	100.0%
		% within Case P100	11.1%	22.0%	20.0%
	More than 10	Count	0	20	20
		% within Duration	.0%	100.0%	100.0%
		% within Case P100	.0%	48.8%	40.0%
Total		Count	9	41	50
		% within Duration	18.0%	82.0%	100.0%
		% within Case P100	100.0%	100.0%	100.0%

P100 VS DURATION

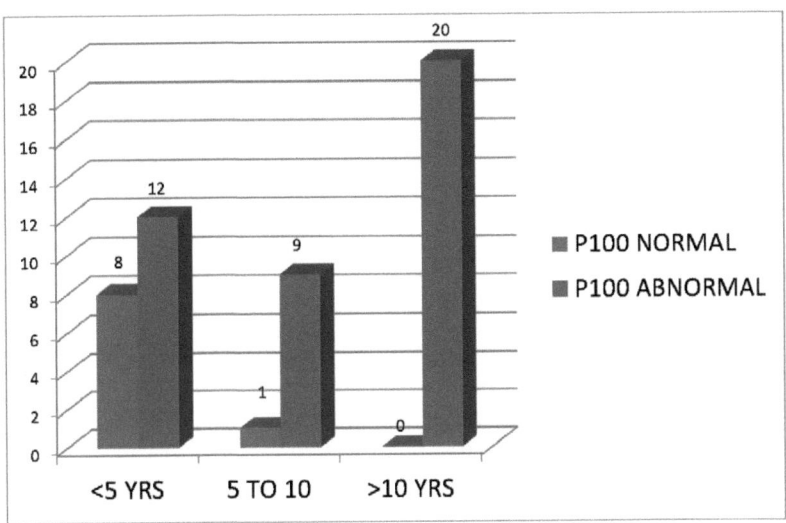

CHART-7: Among those with DM of less than 5 years 8 had normal P100 and 12 had abnormal value, whereas cases with DM more than 10 years all 20 patients had abnormal prolonged P100

P100 VS PNP

PNP * Case P100 Crosstabulation

			Case P100 Normal	Case P100 Abnormal	Total
PNP	No	Count	6	18	24
		% within PNP	25.0%	75.0%	100.0%
		% within Case P100	66.7%	43.9%	48.0%
	Yes	Count	3	23	26
		% within PNP	11.5%	88.5%	100.0%
		% within Case P100	33.3%	56.1%	52.0%
Total		Count	9	41	50
		% within PNP	18.0%	82.0%	100.0%
		% within Case P100	100.0%	100.0%	100.0%

P100 VS PNP

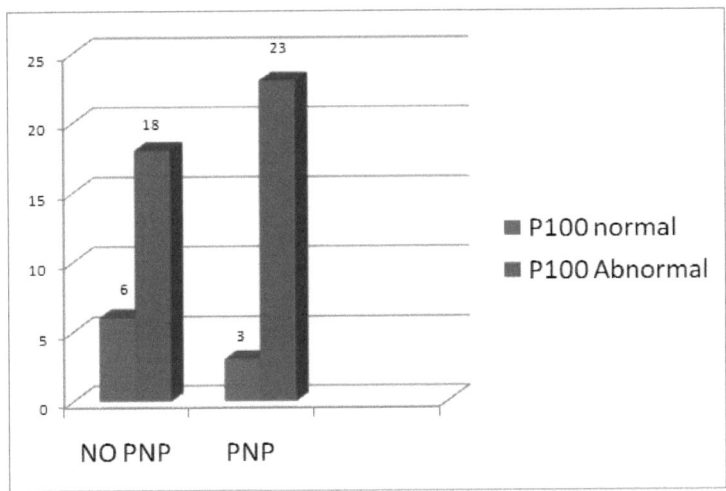

CHART-8: Among cases with PNP 23 had prolonged P100 and 3 had normal P100 whereas those without PNP 18 had prolonged P100 and 6 had normal value.

DISCUSSION

We had 50 cases of diabetes patients who fulfilled the inclusion criteria after vigorously excluding many patients by history, clinical and ophthalmological examination. VEP was done in these 50 patients as well as 50 age and sex matched controls. In VEP there were one positive peak (P100) and two negative peaks (N 70 AND N155). P100 is produced by occipital striate cortex in response to stimulation of visual cortex. P100 is the most prominent wave among all three and is easily reproducible without much variation in an individual. The most ideal parameter in VEP is latency as amplitude has greater variability and is less reliable. Hence we measured P100 latency for all patients.

The mean age our population was 58.44. There were 29 males and 21 females. 7 cases were 40 to 50 years old, 24 between 50 to 60 years and 19 more than 60 years. In our study P100 latencies (ms) was significantly prolonged in diabetics with mean ± SD of (111.24 ± 5.28 ms) as compared to controls (101.30 ± 1.66 ms) with p value <0.003. Among 50 cases 41 cases had prolonged P100 latency when compared to controls only one had P100 prolongation which was statistically very significant. Hence 81% of diabetic patients in our cases had central neuropathy. We also noted that mean prolongation of P100 in cases was much more than in controls.

We further divided the cases into two groups. Those with uncontrolled DM with HbA1c > 7 and those with well controlled DM with HbA1c < 7. Among the 30 cases in uncontrolled group 26 had P100 prolongation and in 20 cases in well controlled group 15 had prolonged P100 latency. 75% of well controlled group and 86% of uncontrolled group had P100 prolongation. There was no statistically significant correlation between the two groups as p value was 0.293. Similarly we looked into duration of DM and classified the cases into 3 groups as <5 years, 5 to 10 years and > 10 years. Among the 20 cases in <5 years group 12 had abnormal P100 and in 5 to 10 year group 9 out of 10 had abnormal P100. In > 10 year group all 20 had prolongation of P100 which was statistically significant (p value <0.03). Hence we noted 100% of cases with >10 year DM had abnormal VEP whereas only 60 % had prolonged P100 in <5 year group.

We also analysed age of patients with P100 latency. We found that 5 out of 7 cases in 40 to 50 year group had abnormal P100. Likewise 18 out of 24 cases in 50 to 60 year group and 18 out of 19 cases in more than 60 year group had prolongation of P100. 71 % of cases between 40 to 50 years, 75 % of cases in 50 to 60 year group and 94 % in more than 60 years group had central neuropathy. There was no statistical significance between age and central neuropathy. We also evaluated peripheral neuropathy (PNP) with central neuropathy and classified the cases into those with PNP and without PNP. Among 24 cases without PNP 18 had prolonged P100 and 23 out of 26 had abnormal P100 in PNP group. 75 % and 94 % of cases had prolonged P100 in the above groups. There was no statistical significance and we found central neuropathy occurring in almost equal percentage in patients with or without PNP.

Similar to our study Dolu H et al, Azal O et al, Szabela D et al, Li P et al, Algan et al, and Comi G et al also concluded prolongation of P100 in diabetic population in their studies. [20,25,23] But Szabela D et al and Algan et al concluded there was no correlation between duration of DM and P100 prolongation.[22] Ziegler et al and Li P et al summarized that P100 prolongation correlated well with glycemic control of DM and even improved with short term glycemic control. [19] We believe that since the sample size was small in most studies and they also included both type 1 and type 2 DM it produced varying results. Moreover in our study 81% of cases had prolonged P100 whereas only 58%, 28 % and 33% of cases had P100 latency abnormality in above studies. In spite of our strict exclusion criteria we produced the maximum percentage of P100 prolongation.

We also believe that inclusion and exclusion criteria varied significantly between each studies resulting in varying percentage of abnormalities in VEP. Our study and Dolu H et al conclude that central neuropathy in DM correlates well with duration of DM and not glycemic control.

At present the significance of P100 prolongation in diabetic patients is not known. It may be due to functional disturbance in visual conduction pathway rather than demyelination or axonal loss. It is also possible that early diabetic preretinopathy due to retinal ganglion cell loss may also contribute to P100 prolongation. Exact pathophysiology for central neuropathy is not known. We suggest it may be multifactorial like PNP both metabolic and vascular factors playing a role. Accumulation of neuropoietic cytokines like TNF-alpha, TGF-beta in visual conduction pathway probably causes delay in P100 latency. As duration of DM increases further accumulation of mediators cause further P100 prolongation.

SUMMARY

- The mean age our population was 58.44

- The P100 latencies (ms) was significantly prolonged in diabetics with mean ± SD of (111.24 ± 5.28 ms) as compared to controls (101.30 ± 1.66 ms) with p value <0.003.

- In our study 81% of diabetic patients in our cases had central neuropathy as evidenced by prolonged P100 latency.

- In cases with DM > 10 years had prolongation of P100 which was statistically significant (p value <0.03).

- There was no statistically significant correlation between P100 and HbA1c or age of patients.

- 75 % of cases without PNP had prolonged P100 and 94 % of cases with PNP had prolonged P100. Although there was no statistical significance, central neuropathy can occur even before PNP.

LIMITATIONS

- Although our sample size is largest when compared to other similar studies we suggest still larger samples are required to validate the findings in our study.

- Many of type 2 DM patients who were above 60 years may have age related changes unrelated to DM causing prolonged P100.

CONCLUSION

- Central neuropathy as measured by P100 latency is very common in type 2 DM.

- Similar to subclinical sensory neuropathy which is detected in majority of DM by nerve conduction studies, subclinical central neuropathy in DM can be detected by VEP.

- It is related to duration of DM and not HbA1c unlike PNP which is related to both.

- Central neuropathy occurs even prior to development of retinopathy or PNP.

- VEP is a non invasive and sensitive screening tool to detect early neurological involvement in DM.

- Since there is a very high incidence of P100 prolongation in DM patients its usefulness in evaluation of multiple sclerosis in a diabetic patient may be limited.

BIBLIOGRAPHY

1. Adams R, Victor M. Brown R. et al. Special Techniques for Neurologic Diagnosis, Adams and Victor's Principles of Neurology - 8th Ed. The McGraw-Hill Companies, Inc.; 2005.

2. Simeon Locke. Nervous System in Diabetes. In Joslin's Diabetes. Lea and Febiger, Philadephia, 1971; 562-4.

3. Michael J.Fowler. Microvasular and macrovascular complications of diabetes.2008;26:1-2.

4. Singh R, Barden A, Mori T, Beilin L. Advanced glycation end products: a review. Diabetologia.2001; 44:129-146.

5. Meier M, King GL. Protein kinase C activation and its pharmacological inhibition in vascular disease. Vasc Med.2000; 5:173-185.

6. Fong DS, Aiello LP, Ferris FL 3RD, Klein R: Diabetic retinopathy. Diabetes care.2004; 27:2540-2553.

7. Gabbay KH. Hyperglycemia, polyol metabolism and complications of diabetes mellitus. Annu Rev Med.1975; 26:521-536.

8. Boulton AJ, Vinik AI, Bril V, Freeman R et al: Diabetic neuropathies: a statement by ADA. Diabetes Care. 2005; 28:956-962.

9. Odom JV, Bach M, Barber C, et al. Visual evoked potentials standard. Documenta Ophthalmologica. 2004;108(2):115–123.

10. Chiappa KH, Yiannikas C. Voluntary alteration of evoked potentials. Ann Neurol 1982; 12:496.

11. Asselman P, Chadwick DW, Marsden CD. Visual evoked responses in diagnosis and management of patients suspected of multiple sclerosis. Brain 1975; 98: 261.

12. Bradley WG, Whitty WM. Acute optic neuritis: its clinical features and their relation to prognosis for recovery of vision. J Neurol Neurosurg Psychiat 1967; 30: 531.

13. Boghen DR, Glaser JS. Ischaemic optic neuropathy. Brain 1975; 98:689.

14. Carroll F. Etiology and treatment of tobacco alcohol amblyopia. Am J Ophthalmol 1974; 47:713.

15. Daneshvar H, Racette L, Coupland SG, et al. Syptomatic and asyptomatic visual loss in patients taking vigabatrin. Ophthalmol 1999; 106:1792.

16. Hennerici M. Dissociated foveal and parafoveal reponses in SACD. Arch Neurol 1985; 42:130.

17. Carroll WM, Kriss A, Baraitser M, et al. The incidence and nature of visual pathway involvement in Friedrich Ataxia. Brain 1980; 103: 413.

18. Bodis-Wollner I. Recovery from cerebral blindness: evoked potential and psychophysical measurements. Clin Neuro-physiol 1977; 42:178.

19. Ziegler O, Guerci B, Algan M, Lonchamp P, Weber M, Drouin P. Improved visual evoked potential latencies in poorly control diabetic patients after short-term strict metabolic control. Diabetes Care 1994. 17:1141-7.

20. Dolu H, Ulas UH, Bolu E, Ozkardes A, Odabasi Z, Ozata M, et al. Evaluation of central neuropathy in type II diabetes mellitus by multimodal evoked potentials. Acta Neurol Belg.2003; 103:206-11.

21. Comi G. Evoked potentials in diabetes mellitus. Clinical Neuroscience. 1997; 4:374.

22. Algan M, Ziegler O et al. Visual evoked potentials in diabetic patients. Diabetes Care 12:227-9, 1989.

23. Szabela DA, Loba J, Pałenga-Pydyn D, Tybor K, Ruxer J, Split W. Klin Oczna. 2005; 107(7-9):492-7.

24. Szabela DA, Loba J, Pałenga-Pydyn D, Tybor K, Ruxer J, Split W. Klin Oczna. 2005; 107(7-9):498-501.

25. Azal O, Ozkardes A, Onde ME, Ozata M, Ozisik G, Corakc A, et al. Visual Evoked Potentials in Diabetic Patients. Tr. J. of Medical Sciences 1998; 28:139-42.

26. Mariani E, Moreo G, Colucci GB. Study of visual evoked potentials in diabetics without retinopathy: correlations with clinical findings and polyneuropathy. Acta Neurologica Scandinavica. 1990;81(4):337–340.

27.Puvanendran K, Devathasan G, Wong PK. Visual evoked responses in diabetes. J. Neurol Neurosurg Psychiatry. 1983; 46:643-7.

28. Yaltkaya K, Balkan S, Baysal AI. Visual evoked potentials in diabetes mellitus. Acta Neurologica Scandinavica. 1988; 77(3):239–241.

29. World Health Organisation Department of Noncommunicable Disease Surveillance (1999). "Definition, Diagnosis and Classification of Diabetes Mellitus and its Complications".

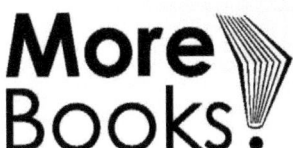
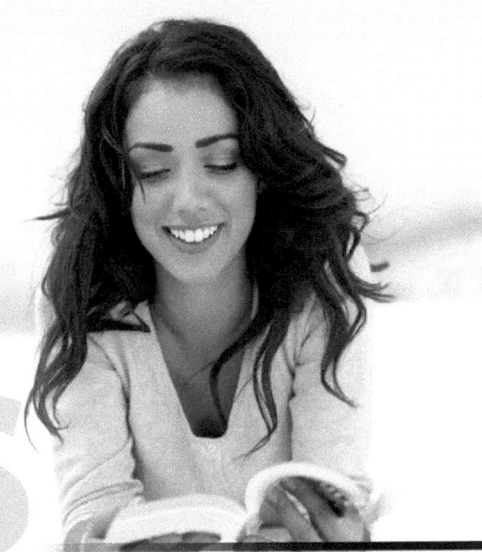 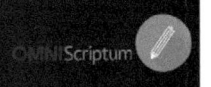

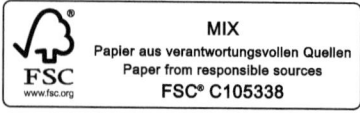